Pressing
RESET
for
Better Breathing

original
strength

Contributors: Sarah Young & Tim Anderson

ISBN: 979-8-9865860-0-7 (Paperback)

How we breathe is how we move through life. How we move is how we breathe. Breathing is movement. Breathing is life.

Breathing is the key that allows us to unlock tension and feel safe. And when we feel safe, it is easier to move past limits. It is easier to heal. It is easier to move through life with power, fluidity, and joy.

No matter what the quality of your breathing is right here, right now in this very moment, there's always room to move from good to better to best.

And as your breathing gets better, all of you gets better. All it takes is the willingness and openness to explore your design, to experience how you were made to breathe and how you were made to move.

This booklet was written to help you do just that.

Our Breathing Design

"Life begins and ends with the exhale."
-Carl Stough (aka Dr. Breath)

The Respiratory Diaphragm

We are designed to breathe with our diaphragms. Breathing with our diaphragms balances us. It grounds us. It allows us to more fully express who we were born to be.

So what is this thing called a diaphragm? It is a dome shaped muscle that caps off the bottom of the ribcage. It separates the torso into the chest and abdomen. It is intricately connected, by fascia and other tissues, to the spine, ribcage, abdominal muscles, internal organs (including the heart), and our nervous system.

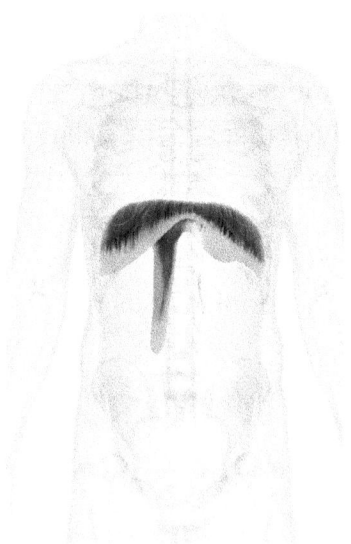

When we breathe with our diaphragms, every part of us is moved.

On the inhale, the diaphragm contracts, glides down the interior of the ribcage, and flattens out. The diaphragm can be thought of as acting like a bellows, creating space and pulling air into the lungs.

When we exhale, it glides back up the interior of the ribcage, riding the lungs in order to aid them in emptying, returning to its domed shape.

And the exhale, well, the exhale is where the magic happens. Inhalation is simply a reflex.

When we allow a generous exhale, our ability to take air in - our inhalation reflex - improves and our diaphragm can grow stronger. We can grow stronger.

Along with moving air in and out of the lungs, the diaphragm acts as a pump to help circulate blood, lymphatic fluid, and cerebral spinal fluid.

Diaphragmatic breathing also dynamically balances our nervous system.

Once again, when we breathe as we're designed to breathe, every part of us is moved.

The Rib Cage

The rib cage offers structure and protection to the lungs, the heart, and other vital organs.

There are twelve pairs of ribs. All rib pairs join with the thoracic spine in the back and all but two pairs have connections to the sternum in the front.

There are 37 bones in the rib cage which interact to form approximately 100 joints. And joints are made for movement.

The more we breathe according to our design, the more these joints can move. And the more freely the rib cage can move, the better we can breathe.

In between the ribs are intercostal muscles which aid the ribs in moving as we exhale and inhale.

The Lungs

Our lungs are designed to be spongy, elastic, and slippery. This allows the lungs to change in size as we breathe and allows them to glide within the rib cage.

When we inhale, the lungs inflate much like balloons. When we exhale, air is released from the lungs and they return to their resting volume.

Air breathed in through the nose travels down the throat and into airways that branch out into each lung. At the ends of these branches, inside of the lungs, are tiny air sacs called alveoli. The alveoli are where the lungs and blood exchange oxygen and carbon dioxide.

Nasal Breathing

We are designed to breathe nasally. Nasal breathing aids diaphragmatic function.

Inhaling nasally preps the air for our lungs by filtering, warming, and humidifying the air.

Inhaling nasally also produces NO (nitric oxide) in the nasal passages. NO has been found to be a frontline of defense against airborne bacteria. It also aids the delivery of oxygen (O_2) to tissues and reduces blood pressure.

Exhaling through the nose allows air to leave the body more slowly, which aids the body in balancing levels of O_2 and CO_2.

Exhaling through the nose also helps to keep the body hydrated.

Please don't overthink nasal breathing. Mouth breathing happens and can be useful. It's just not meant to be our default way of breathing.

The Power of the Tongue and a Smile

Allowing the tongue to rest on the roof of the mouth supports head control, which assists in opening airways. It also improves access to the respiratory diaphragm.

Smiling helps to open the airways too.

When we breathe nasally, diaphragmatically, and with a smile, we prime our bodies for optimal breathing, which primes our bodies for optimal movement.

Breathing Outside Our Design

We have muscles in our upper chest, shoulders, neck, and low back that can assist the diaphragm with breathing. These accessory breathing muscles are designed to help out when we're under threat or think we're under threat - when we don't feel safe.

When these muscles go from assisting to driving the breath, the result is excess tension in these same muscles and the rest of the body. Our breathing default then switches to a tension inducing state. It keeps us in a dis-stressed state of fight/freeze/flight. It keeps us in a state of feeling unsafe.

Add to this modern life's own unique challenges. We tend to sit more and move less. We stare at screens a lot. We forget how to move with gravity, and instead gravity compresses us.

As a result, our bodies become tense, tight, and achy. This adds to our dis-stress and throws us further off our breathing game. We then lose out on the benefits that come from diaphragmatic breathing.

But we don't have to stay stuck in this stressed way of being. We can toggle the switch on our nervous system from a dis-stressed (sympathetic) state of breathing and being to a relaxed (parasympathetic) state of breathing and being.

And each of us has this internal toggle switch, this reset button.

Using it can restore you to the relaxed state in which your body, mind, and spirit are able to feel safe and heal. And from that space you are able to flow and move past limits.

All you have to do is Press RESET.

How You can Press RESET

You were born with a reset button you can utilize to restore your breathing, your nervous system, your body, all of you. And this reset button isn't a hack. It isn't a mystery. It is wired into each of us. It's simply (and powerfully) a part of who you are.

To utilize this reset button, all you need to do is engage in the Three Pillars of Human Movement. It really is that simple. It really is that easy.

The Three Pillars of Human Movement

We were all born with movement pillars that were designed to allow us to express ourselves without limits:

1. Breathe with the diaphragm.
2. Activate the vestibular system.
3. Engage in contra-lateral movement patterns (your gait pattern).

Engaging in these three movement pillars serves you by nourishing your nervous system, which allows you to express more of your reflexive strength, resilience, and healing.

These movement pillars reconnect you with how you were designed to move through the world and can be easily expressed through these five developmental movement patterns you engaged in as a child:

1. Breathing
2. Head control
3. Rolling
4. Rocking
5. Crawling

As you Press RESET with the movement resets in this booklet, please stay curious. Feel how your body feels. Notice with a sense of wonder. Stay within a comfortable range of motion.

Now let's look at how each of these movement patterns can help you Press RESET on your breathing.

Pressing
RESET

Reset 1

Breathing

"Breathing is the balance wheel of the body."
-Jessica Wolf

Yes, Pressing RESET on your breathing is the place to start reclaiming more of your breathing potential and more of your movement potential. Because breathing is the foundation of all movement, it enriches all the other resets and benefits from all the other resets. Breathing balances us.

It can be helpful to initiate the process of Pressing RESET with breathing with a slow exhale out. The exhale is what allows your body's inhalation reflex to fire.

Allowing exhalation to be fully but not forcefully expressed helps you hone your inhalation reflex. It creates space for you to breathe whole breaths instead of partial, shallow breaths.

Tongue placement is important. Gently rest the tip of your tongue on the roof of your mouth slightly behind your front teeth.

Once you've exhaled through your nose; slowly, quietly, deeply, and fluidly, "listen" for your body to say, "it's time to breathe in." That's the inhalation reflex.

When that happens simply breathe in. Allow yourself to feel the coolness of the air as it enters your nose and spreads across your sinuses.

Imagine filling your lungs from the bottom to the top as if your lungs are two big balloons. As you do this you'll feel your belly rise and your ribcage open to create space for your lungs as they inflate.

As you inhale, explore sensing your back spreading through its width and your spine lengthening as your ribcage gently swings open.

On the exhale, simply allow it to happen. Exhale slowly and quietly through your nose. No need to force the air out. In fact, forcing air in or out gets in the way of breathing.

Then after an easy exhale simply wait for the inhalation reflex and breathe in.

With each breath, let go of any tension you no longer need.

Let's explore a few breathing positions to start with the understanding that different positions and movements require different things from your breathing.

And please know that this booklet only shows a few of the many possible Original Strength resets available to you.

Breathing Resets

**"We aren't designed to breathe.
We are designed to be breathed."**

-Jean McClelland

Movement #1

SUPINE BELLY BREATHING

Lie on your back with your knees bent, feet on the floor. If need be you can place a thin pillow under your head for comfort. This position allows your body to be fully supported by the surface you're on. You might place one hand lightly on your chest and the other hand lightly on your abdomen just below your navel. Simply feel your body move under your hands. Allow your breath to move like a wave. Breathe in this position for a few minutes. Sense your breath as it moves out and in.

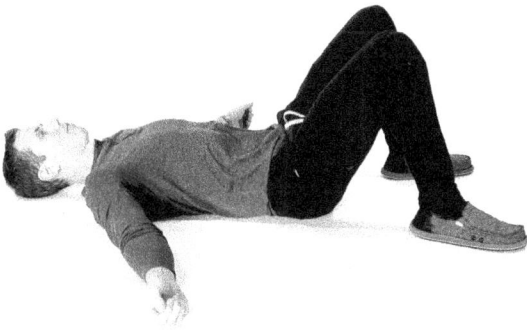

Movement #2

CROCODILE BREATHING

Lie on your stomach with your forehead resting on the backs of your hands. In this position your body is once again supported, and you get sensory feedback from the surface you're on. Gravity works on your body a bit differently than in the first position. Breathe in this position for a few minutes. Notice how your breath feels as you exhale and inhale.

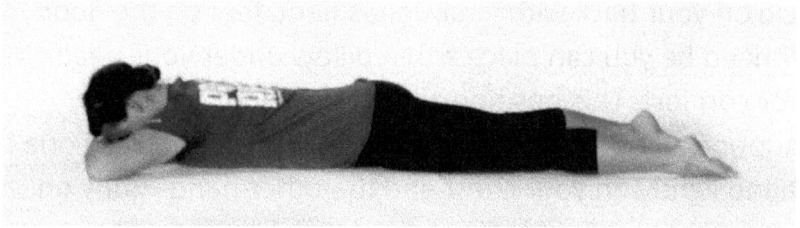

Movement #3

SEATED QUADRUPED

Begin in a quadruped position on hands and knees. Gently shift your weight back to sit on your heels and slide your hands closer to your knees, eyes gazing softly on the horizon, chest gently lifted. More of your weight will be on your heels. Relax in this position. You may use a pillow or rolled up towel between your butt and heels for comfort. As always, remember tongue placement.

And yes, gravity will act on your body differently in this position. Feel your breath as it moves out and in.

*While not pictured, you might also explore breathing by sitting in a chair, bent forward (hinged) at hips, with hands or forearms on thighs.

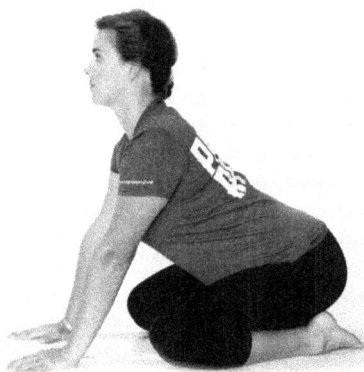

Breathing Within the Resets

"Smile, breathe and go slowly."

-Thich Nhat Hanh

As you move through the following resets, it can be helpful to go slowly in order to explore your breathing within the resets .

Check in with your breathing. Is it more or less challenging to breathe whole breaths in some resets than others? Simply sense and notice.

Explore how your movement within the resets shifts as you mindfully focus on the reset of breathing.

Pause at points within a reset to Press RESET with breathing. Are you able to breathe with the same fluidity you did with the stand alone breathing resets?

If you sense a sticky spot, or your body's tension level jumps at points during a reset, try pausing at those points and Press RESET with breathing.

Be curious but judgment free. Feel and sense.

And remember, it's all about good, better, best.

Some breathing points to remember:

- Keep your tongue on the roof of your mouth with mouth gently closed. Jaw relaxed. Breathe nasally.
- Exhale fully but without force. Then pause for your body to say, "it's time to breathe." Then inhale (inhalation is a reflex).
- Inhale generously through your nose. Feel the coolness of the air as it moves through your nose, across your sinuses, and into your lungs.
- Breathe into the width and length of your back all the way up to your armpits.
- Repeat the cycle. Breathe slowly, fluidly, and quietly, allowing yourself to feel greater ease with each breath.

Reset 2

Head Control Resets

Pressing RESET with head control is important because it activates your vestibular system. Your vestibular system is your balance system and a sensory information collection point. This helps you get your head on straight so that your head is more reflexively balanced over your body, allowing your airway to be more optimally positioned for breathing.

Head control resets also offer tension relief for tight neck muscles, helping to restore optimal neck function. This allows for better air flow and circulation of all kinds.

Movement #1

SUPINE HEAD CONTROL

Lie on your back with knees to chest (or knees bent and feet on the floor). This position allows your body to be fully supported by the surface you're on.

Head rotations: In this position you'll look to the right with your eyes and allow your head to follow. Then you'll look left with your eyes and allow your head to follow with ease. Eyes softly lead the head. Head follows. Rotate your head, gently, side to side. Repeat 5 to 10 times.

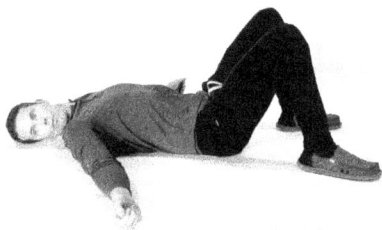

Head nods: In this position, with your head supported by the floor, you'll nod up and down. Eyes look up, then your head nods up. Eyes look down and head nods down. Gently tuck your chin. At the end of the nod down you can lift your head off the floor (as in photo) or not. If you lift your head keep your chin gently tucked as you lower your head to the floor to begin your next nod up. Repeat 5 to 10 times.

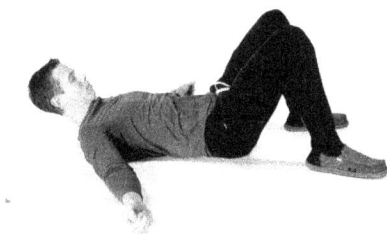

Movement #2

TV WATCHING POSITION

Lying on your stomach, gently lift your chest and support yourself on your forearms. In this position your body is once again supported (mostly) by the surface you're on.

Head rotations: Perform 5 to 10 head rotations looking over each shoulder as far as you can. Eyes lead. Head follows. Allow your body to respond.

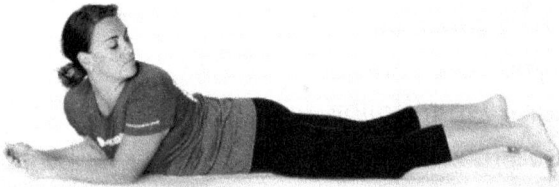

Head nods: Perform 5 to 10 head nods. This will be similar to the supine position, but gravity will act differently on your body. Eyes lead. Head follows. Allow your body to respond.

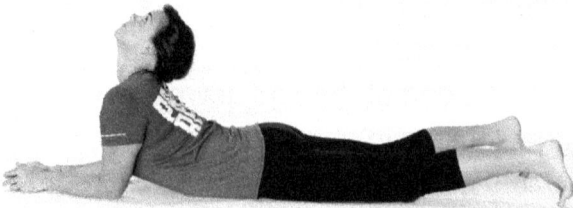

Movement #3

SEATED QUADRUPED

Begin in a quadruped position on hands and knees. Gently shift your weight back to sit on your heels and slide your hands closer to your knees, eyes on the horizon, chest gently lifted. Relax in this position, using a pillow or rolled up towel between your butt and heels for comfort if needed.

Head rotations: Perform 5 to 10 head rotations. Eyes lead. Head follows. Body responds.

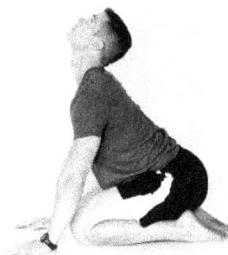

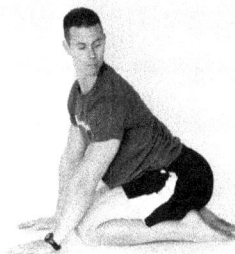

Head nods: Perform 5 to 10 head nods. Eyes lead. Head follows. Body responds.

*While not pictured, you might also explore head control resets by sitting in a chair, bent forward (hinged) at hips, with hands or forearms on thighs.

Remember, at any point during head control reset, if you feel your body resist the movement, try Pressing RESET with your breathing.

Rolling Resets

Rolling also stimulates the vestibular system. It provides a sensory rich experience and soothes the nervous system.

Rolling is a great way to open up the thoracic spine and the ribcage. Both often become locked down due to too much sitting and too little movement. Mental and emotional stress can also rob these areas of freedom to move.

And remember, there are approximately 100 joints in the ribcage. Rolling is a wonderful way to gently remind the thoracic spine and ribcage how they're made to move.

Rolling sets the ribcage free to dance more fluidly with the diaphragm and lungs for more optimal breathing.

Movement #1

EGG ROLL

Lie on your back with knees to chest. Gently place your hands on your shins. Lead the roll with your eyes by looking to the right then allow your head to gently rotate to the right to follow your eyes. Keep looking as far to the right as you can and allow your body to follow. Then look to the left with your eyes, turn your head gently to the left, and allow your body to roll to the left. Pause at points in the roll when you feel your body resist the roll. Press RESET with your breathing at those points. It's ok if you can only roll in a small range of motion to start. Roll back and forth this way for a couple of minutes. Feel free to roll longer if you like.

Eyes lead. Head follows. Body responds.

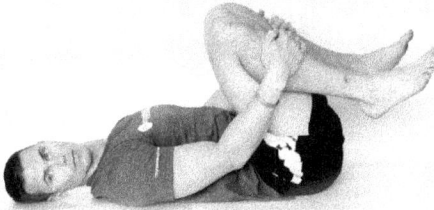

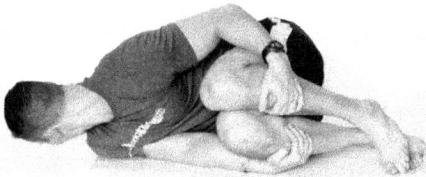

Movement #2

ELBOW ROLL

Lie on your belly with arms comfortably over your head and legs extended. Slightly bend your right elbow and reach for the floor behind you. Pause at points in the roll when you feel your body resist the roll. Press RESET with your breathing at those points. Stay within a comfortable range of motion. Repeat on the left side. Keep your arms and legs relaxed. Roll this way for a couple of minutes, more if you like.

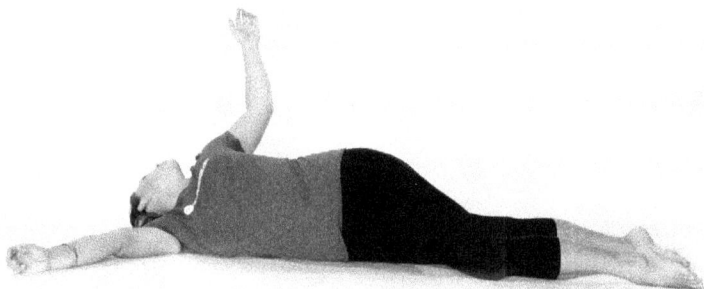

Movement #3

SUPINE LOWER BODY HALF ROLL

Lie on your back with arms comfortably over your head and legs extended. Gently bend your right leg and bring it to your chest. Gently reach your knee across your opposite hip as if you're trying to touch the floor with your knee. Keep the leg bent and relaxed. Pause at points in the roll when you feel your body resist the roll. Press RESET with your breathing at those points. Stay within a comfortable range of motion. Repeat on the left side. Keep your arms and legs relaxed. Roll this way for a couple of minutes or more.

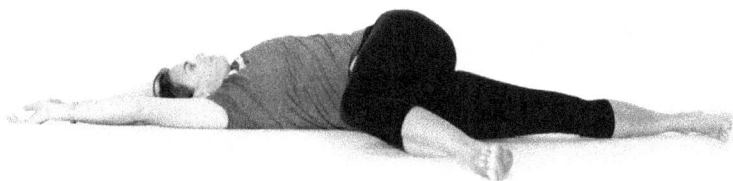

Rocking Resets

Rocking is gentle strength training for the whole body. Rocking is where the body learns to move with gravity rather than be compressed and beaten down by it. When we get on our hands and knees, our body's stabilizers learn to stabilize and our prime movers learn how to get us moving.

Rocking both stimulates the vestibular system and soothes the nervous system. Rocking integrates the joints of the body and prepares the shoulders and hips for crawling, walking, and running. Rocking also restores posture.

Rocking offers unique challenges for breathing. It teaches the diaphragm how it can move while the rest of the body is either stabilizing or moving.

Movement #1

ROCKING ON HANDS AND KNEES

Begin on your hands and knees. Sense your body balanced over your hands and knees. Remember tongue position with mouth gently closed. Head up. Eyes on the horizon. Chest is gently lifted (sternum up), and the lower back is relaxed and flat. Feel what it feels like to breathe in this quadruped position. Now rock by shifting your weight over your hands then back over your feet. Repeat, going back and forth. Keep your back relaxed and flat and don't let it round up or bow up as you rock. Feel how your breath shifts as you rock. Breathe at sticky points. Rock back and forth for a couple of minutes, more if you like.

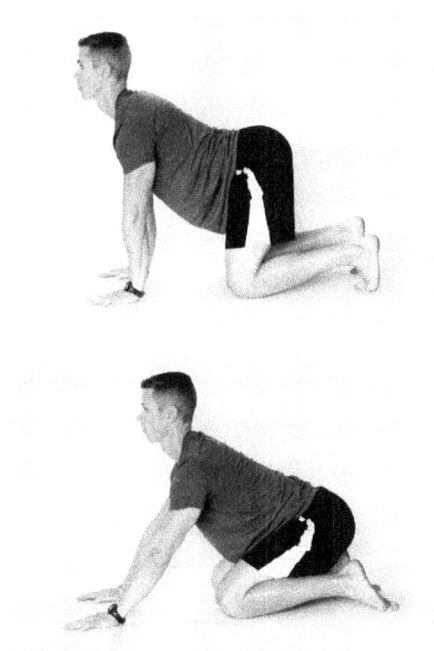

Movement #2

ROCKING WITH ONE ARM RAISED

This rocking position will require a bit more from your body and your breathing, as you'll have a smaller base of support. Begin as you did in the hands and knees rocking position. Extend your right arm in front of you. Rock in this position for 30 seconds to a minute. Then do the same with your left arm raised. Repeat for a few cycles.

Are you able to keep your breathing fluid like a wave? What do you notice about how your body responds with one arm lifted versus the other arm lifted?

*Feet can be in plantar flexion (laces down) or dorsiflexion (toes under) when rocking or crawling.

Crawling Resets

Crawling strengthens and nourishes the nervous system. It connects both halves of the brain together, making it healthier and more efficient. It integrates sensory systems with the vestibular system.

Crawling reflexively connects the body and ties it together. It reflexively strengthens the body, making it easier to move more fluidly with grace and power. It sharpens the body's postural reflex, allowing it to be more optimally expressed.

Crawling is where the diaphragm learns how to work within the gait pattern. It's a gentle way to reconnect the diaphragm with how it's designed to move during movements such as walking and running.

Movement #1

HANDS AND KNEES CRAWLING

Begin on your hands and knees. Sense your body balanced over your hands and knees. Remember tongue position with mouth gently closed. Head up. Eyes softly on the horizon. Chest is gently lifted (sternum up), and the lower back is relaxed and flat. Feel what it feels like to breathe in this quadruped position. Begin crawling by moving opposite arms and legs together. Play with crawling forward and backward for a few minutes or more. Press RESET with your breathing at different points in your crawl stride.

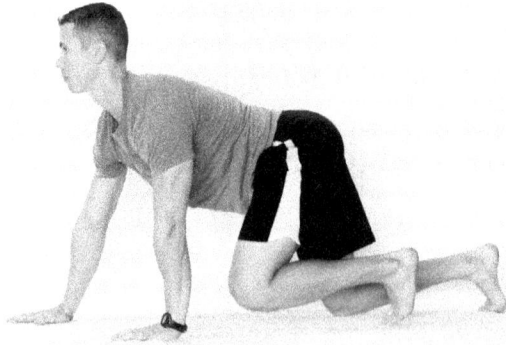

Movement #2

SPEED SKATERS

Begin on your hands and knees. Sense your body balanced over your hands and knees. Remember tongue position with mouth gently closed. Breathe nasally. Head up. Eyes on the horizon. Chest is gently lifted (sternum up), and the lower back is relaxed and flat. Feel what it feels like to breathe in this quadruped position. Lift the opposite arm and leg back at the same time. Do 10 speed skaters on each side. Press RESET with your breathing at different points in the speed skater reset.

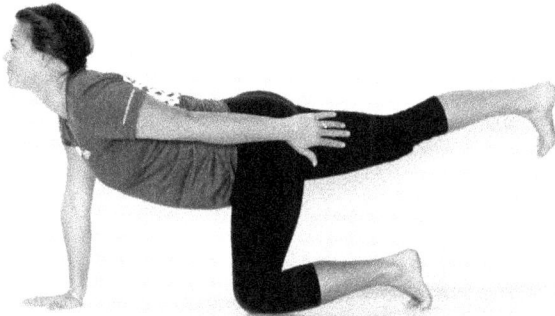

Movement #3

CROSS-CRAWLS

Stand up and sense your
body balanced over your feet.
Remember tongue position with
mouth gently closed. Breathe
nasally. Head up. Eyes on the
horizon. Feel what it feels
like to breathe in this upright
position. Touch your opposite
limbs together. You can touch
the hand to the thigh, elbow to
knee, etc. Press RESET with your
breathing at different points
during cross-crawls. Play with
cross-crawls for a few minutes
or longer if you prefer.

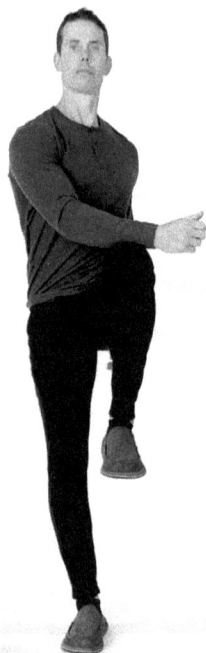

Do not dismiss the simplicity
of this movement. This movement can be the easiest and
most effective entry point that begins the restoration
and strengthening of the nervous system. Cross-crawls
can help nourish and rewire the brain by tapping into
and making the most of its neuroplasticity. It can serve
a person in learning and even overcoming challenges
in learning. Cross-crawls set the body free to move and
express itself.

The Power in Your Design

The power of movement restoration, the hope of healing, and the expression of strength all live in your nervous system. Breathing balances your nervous system so that healing and strength can flow more freely. Your very design contains the movement program intended to keep you strong, able, and healthy. Breathing is the key that unlocks the power of your design.

Spending just a few minutes every day, relearning or remembering how to do these movements will enable you to live your life better - with strength and health.

Your body truly is awesomely and wonderfully made. It is designed to be strong and able, always. Everything you need to experience this is inside your nervous system, waiting for you to breathe and move with it. In other words, your Original Strength is inside. It's your move...

Creating a Breathing Reset Practice

"Start where you are. Use what you have. Do what you can."

-Arthur Ashe

Breathing is nothing short of a miracle. And the more you embrace how you are designed to breathe, the more you can express the greater miracle that is you.

The place to start is right where you are, with a daily breathing practice. This will require you making time for you. Please know you are more than worth that investment.

You might begin with two, three to five minute sessions: one in the morning when you wake up to begin your day refreshed, and one before bed so that you'll be more relaxed and ready for sleep.

You could do a mix of resets, utilizing the ones presented in this booklet. The possibilities are endless.

Three Minute Example

Choose a comfortable position.

One minute: Do a breathing reset presented in this booklet
One minute: Do some head control resets as presented in this booklet
One minute: Do rolling or rocking resets as presented in this booklet.

If you have more time, perhaps you can create space in your day for a 10 minute session or two. Simply use the resets in this booklet and explore.

You might also do breathing check-ins with yourself as you move through your day. This could take the form of three mindful breaths before you eat a meal.

You could also take a mindful breath or two at other points during your day: before you start or pick up your device(s), before a meeting, while waiting in the check out line, while you cook, during your daily chores, while reading, as you knit, between sets at the gym, during transit, before you begin your workday, at the end of your workday — anytime is a good time to check in and Press RESET with breathing. Doing so makes everything better, including you.

Want to learn more?

This booklet was designed to give a brief overview of the Original Strength System and how it can help you Press RESET on your breathing.

We put it together because we know it can help everyone and anyone. If you do nothing more than what is in this booklet, you will notice many changes in how your mind and body begin to feel.

Original Strength is a human movement education company with a mission to transform the world by teaching people to move better, so they can live life better.

We do this by conducting courses that train and certify coaches, instructors, and individuals. We also develop educational materials for PE and K-12 teachers, physical therapy and other medical professionals, fitness/health & wellness instructors, sports conditioning professionals, and individuals/groups working with vestibular and neuromuscular functionality.

If you want to know more about Pressing RESET and regaining your Original Strength, visit https://originalstrength.net. There you will find a variety of books, free video tutorials (OS Movement Snax), and a complete listing of our courses and OS Certified Professionals near you.

You may want to consider finding an OS Certified Professional. An OS Certified Professional can take you through an Original Strength Screen and Assessment (OSSA) which is the quickest and easiest way to pinpoint the best starting point for you to begin Pressing RESET in order for you to reclaim your original strength. They can also work with you as you move forward on your journey to help you get the most out of your body.

We encourage you to reach out to the OS team with any questions you may have. Keep us updated with your progress or tell us your story at Progress@OriginalStrength.net or MyStory@OriginalStrength.net.

Acknowledgment

We would like to acknowledge the work and inspiration of the following teachers who seek to help others return to their natural way of breathing. Their works and words have been a source of inspiration for this booklet.

Lynn Martin
Jean McClelland
Jessica Wolf
Master Wasentha Young

Press RESET now and live life better because you were awesomely and wonderfully made to accomplish amazing things.

For more information:

⏻riginal
strength

Original Strength Systems, LLC
OriginalStrength.net

PressingRESETfor@Originalstrength.net

original
strength

originalstrength.net

Published by

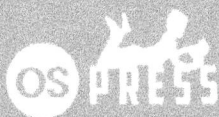